I0486154

Taking the FEAR Out of Knee Replacement Surgery

Top 5 Fears Examined and Explained

By Dr. Melody Stevens, PT, DPT

Taking the FEAR Out of Knee Replacement Surgery - Top 5 Fears Examined and Explained

Copyright © 2015 by Onward Physical Therapy and Wellness Center, Inc.

All rights reserved. No part of this book may be reproduced or transmitted in any form or by any means without written permission from the author.

Printed in USA by CreateSpace (www.createspace.com)

Dedication

This book is dedicated to my amazing husband Matt, and my supportive family. Their encouragement and excitement as I pursue my goals is the most amazing blessing anyone could ask for.

A special thank you to Henry Evans and Kat Loterzo for your inspiration, support and business savvy to help make my dreams a reality.

John 3:16

Table of Contents

Preface

Thank you for purchasing or reading my very first printed book! As I write this, I'm sharing with you my eight years of education coupled with seven years of in-field experience to bring you this first printed endeavor.

By working closely with my patients, their families, caregivers and surgeons, this guide is primed to give you both insight and expertise on what the patient will go through when getting a knee replacement.

As a healthcare professional and successful entrepreneur, my experiences of owning my own clinic, working in world renowned hospitals and even working directly in my patient's homes have given me the perfect view of all the pieces of the puzzle you're going through or might encounter.

It's my joy to make YOUR life easier, and everything I do and the resources I create are all based around that.

I realized awhile back that only working in ONE city, with only ONE clinic and being only ONE person was NOT going meet my internal desire to HELP MORE PEOPLE!

Hence, I'm entering the world via books, e-books, instructional videos, articles, resources, social media and the like, to make a bigger impact on more people's lives.

And I hope you'll be one of them!

To learn how to work with me to have the best recovery you can after your knee replacement surgery, visit BestKneeRecovery.com

Here's to your best knees,

~Dr. Melody

Introduction

In this book you'll find the Top 5 Fears that most people face when considering knee replacement surgery.

I explain each fear through the eyes of the patient and help to explain, inform and educate you on the various concerns and "unknowns" that most people are just thrown into, before they have the whole picture or know what's next.

I've also include practical action steps, worksheets and cheat-sheets to help you lay out your concerns and have a concise and clear picture of the situation so you're set up for success *before* the actual surgery.

Now get to reading so we can start squashing your fears, one by one! Enjoy.

<u>Tackling Fear #1</u>

Fear of the Recovery Process

Now let's face it, you've probably had a friend or two already go through this surgery, and you've most likely **heard their discomforts** about the rehab they had to go through and the many hours in physical therapy, so are you *really* up for all that?

Is it *really* worth the hours in therapy and the healing process to justify the reward in the *end?*

The short answer: **YES!**

As a Doctor of Physical Therapy I've worked with patients on every aspect of this process from strength training with pre-op jitters, to fresh out of the operating room, then in-home therapy right after the hospital, and finally in the outpatient clinic for the final stages of rehab.

I've seen it all: the good, the bad, and the ugly. And yes, it can get ugly. BUT, those cases are few and far between, and most often it's from poor rehab on the patient's part, not for lack of skill and training from the surgeons and therapists.

So therefore, more often than not, *you* **can control the destiny** of your ultimate **triumphant recovery!**

I'd be lying if I said it was easy and pain-free, but sadly, *I cannot tell a lie.*

But what I *can* tell you is that with proper rehab instruction and unwavering dedication on your end, **the recovery process is not something to fear, but something to conquer!**

<u>Tackling Fear #2</u>

Fear of the Risk Factors

Every major undertaking has it's fair share of risks.

Be it in business, your personal life or in healthcare. But more often than not, the **benefits of success far outweigh the possibilities of risk.**

But let's get down to it.

What *are* the risks for a knee replacement surgery?
- -Complication with prosthetic implant
- -Blood clot (DVT) or hematoma
- -Cardiac complications
- -Post-op infection
- -Complication of surgical incision
- -Respiratory complication

Ok.

Well at least we've laid them out.

The **good news** is that recent studies show **only 7.5%** of 1.82 million patients had a complication on that list. *Less than* 1 out of 10!

This is why so many precautions are taken *before* surgery to make sure your body is prepared for the best outcome of successfully avoiding any complications.

Knee replacement surgeries are becoming more common, and therefore surgeons and medical device companies **continue to improve** on their speed and efficiency to get you in and out of the operating room as quickly and safely as possible.

And in case you didn't know, you'll already be up and walking the hallways in your hospital gown *only a few hours after surgery!*

Now that we've outlined the negatives, let's take a look at a small sampling of the **boundless positives** this surgery provides!

    ✓   Arthritic pain relief! (This deserves multiple spots on this list!)

- ✓ Improved mobility in and out of your home
- ✓ Return to activity and recreation
- ✓ Regained sense of self and independence
- ✓ Extended years on the golf course, swimming pool, tennis court

You get the idea. :)

In fact, in the same report I mentioned earlier, **9 out of 10 patients experienced dramatic pain relief,** and **95%** report they were satisfied with their procedure.

On the next page is an awesome graphic to point out some of the highlights and current stats about knee replacements in the U.S. as of 2012.

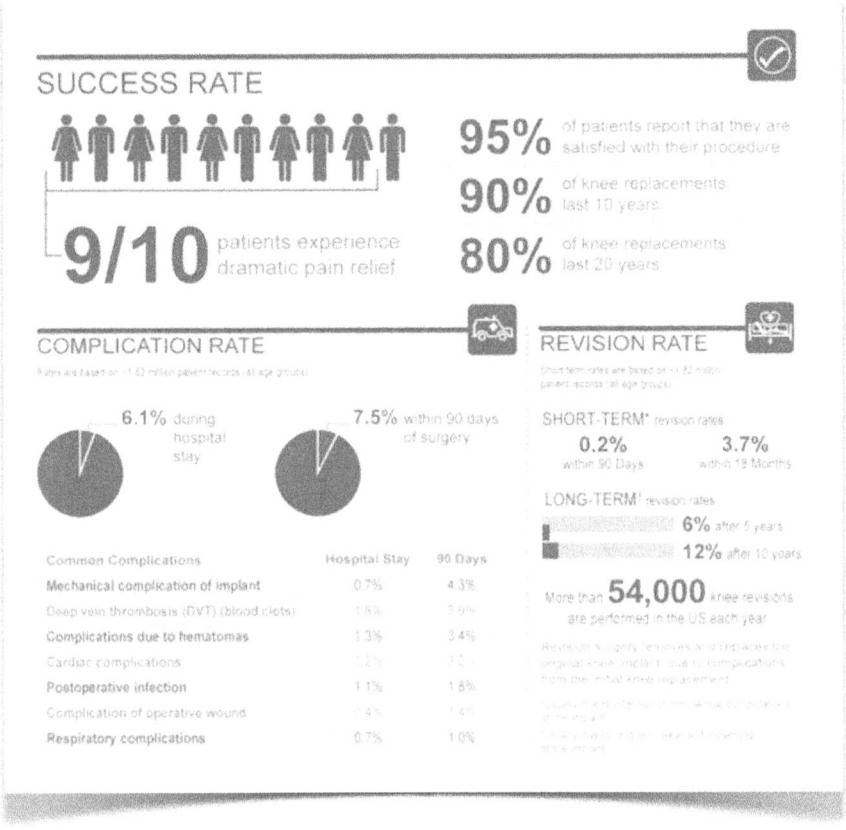

SUCCESS RATE

95% of patients report that they are satisfied with their procedure

90% of knee replacements last 10 years

9/10 patients experience dramatic pain relief

80% of knee replacements last 20 years

COMPLICATION RATE

Rates are based on 1.82 million patient records (all age groups)

6.1% during hospital stay

7.5% within 90 days of surgery

Common Complications	Hospital Stay	90 Days
Mechanical complication of implant	0.7%	4.3%
Deep vein thrombosis (DVT) (blood clots)	1.5%	3.9%
Complications due to hematomas	1.3%	3.4%
Cardiac complications	1.2%	3.2%
Postoperative infection	1.1%	1.8%
Complication of operative wound	0.4%	1.4%
Respiratory complications	0.7%	1.0%

REVISION RATE

Short-term rates are based on 1.82 million patient records (all age groups)

SHORT-TERM* revision rates

0.2% within 90 Days

3.7% within 18 Months

LONG-TERM† revision rates

6% after 5 years

12% after 10 years

More than **54,000** knee revisions are performed in the US each year

Revision surgery removes and replaces the original knee implant due to complications from the initial knee replacement.

Courtesy of Health Line Networks and PearlDiver Technologies.

As you can see, **9 out of 10** in _1.82 million people_ experienced dramatic pain relief after surgery, and **95% were satisfied** with their procedure.

The rewards really *can* outweigh the risks.

Tackling Fear #3

Fear of Outliving the Prosthetic

Alright. We can't deny that life expectancies continue to go up
as modern medicine advances, so the question then remains,

> *"If I need a knee replacement at 60, but I'm going to live well into my 80's or 90's, do I really want to (and will I be healthy enough to) go through another surgery 20 years from now?"*

Valid concern.

The more important question to be asking is,

> *"If I live another 20 or 30 years, will I really be able to enjoy those years if I*

continue to <u>suffer</u> with my current knee pain?"

Now it becomes an issue of your quality of life.

This is when I think it becomes necessary to make an **Pros and Cons** list to help you be more objective.

Try to take a step back and look at the **big picture.**

I've provided a template for you on the next page. **Photocopy and enlarge it,** *and get to work!*

Or you can visit
http://www.SuperiorKneeRehab.com/?p=367
and **print it out full page!**

"To Have, Or Not To Have, Knee Replacement Surgery... That is the Question"

Pros	Cons

Circle your answers to the categories below about your *current situation*:

Pain level *(0 is no pain, 10 is intolerable):* 0 1 2 3 4 5 6 7 8 9 10

Current activity/mobility level: Poor   Fair   Good   Excellent

Recreational activities: Poor   Fair   Good   Excellent

Independence level: Poor   Fair   Good   Excellent

Quality of life *(1 is very poor, 10 is excellent):* 1 2 3 4 5 6 7 8 9 10

© 2015 SuperiorKneeRehab.com

List the <u>Pros</u>

Under the <u>Pros</u> side start listing all the things you can foresee in the next 20-30 years that may take place for you personally and professionally that you want to be able to participate in and fully enjoy.

(examples: grandchildren's weddings, upcoming vacations, family reunions, charity functions etc.)

List the <u>Cons</u>

Under the <u>Cons</u> side list all of the things that you're hesitant and fearful of and consequences that may occur that would deter you from having the surgery.

Lastly, rate your current levels of ability.
In the following categories to get a good picture of your present situation.

- Pain level (0-10, 0 is no pain, 10 is intolerable)
- Current activity/mobility level (Poor, Fair, Good, Excellent)
- Recreational activities (Poor, Fair, Good, Excellent)

- Independence level (Poor, Fair, Good, Excellent)
- Quality of life score (1-10, 1 is very poor, 10 is excellent)

I'll wait for you while you get that done.

Once you're through, I'll see you right back here. :)

Done?

Ok great!

Now that you have a more defined and overall picture of your current state and a better outlining of the pros and cons you're facing, that should help to **put your mind at ease** or at least have more clarity.

Regardless if you decide to have your knee replacement surgery or not, we've got ways to help you live better and with less pain.

Final food for thought:

In the article I mentioned previously about risk factors, you'll be happy to know that **90% of knee replacements lasted 10 years, and 80% lasted *20 years!***

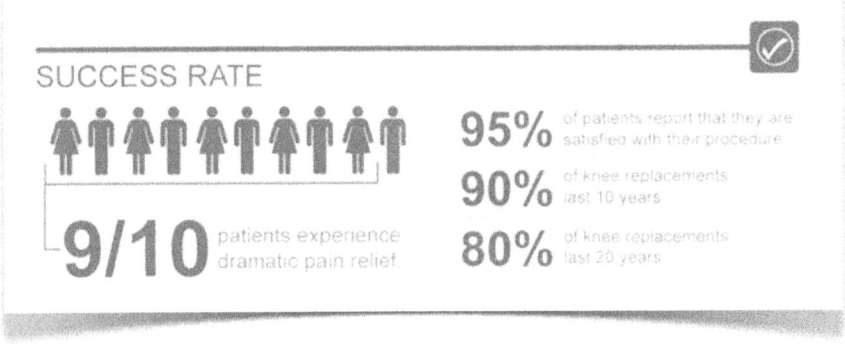

Courtesy of Health Line Networks and PearlDiver Technologies.

Tackling Fear #4

Fear of Burdening Friends and Family for Help

No one wants to be a burden.

I get it.

So how much help will you *actually* need?

What can you do to be the most **prepared ahead of time** to lessen the demand on others?

Let's take a look methodically through the process of getting knee replacement surgery, and break it down from there.

Of course you *could* have help with everything, from housecleaning to bathing, if you wanted it, or if you it was offered to you, but let's go from the perspective that you're **going 100% solo** on this journey.

Pre-Surgery

Others: Transportation to hospital (Worst case scenario you can look into medical transport services in your area, or go by taxi or public transportation)

Others	Self
✓ Transportation to Hospital	✓ Home Safety Preparation
	✓ Meal Prep

Self: Home safety prep and pre-made meals for once you're home.

This would include removing throw rugs and clearing hallways and high traffic pathways (especially to the bathroom and kitchen), and installation of grab bars in bathroom and shower, if needed.

And thinking of meal-prep that you can do ahead of time would be things that can be frozen ahead of time for easy cooking afterward.

Since most people are in the hospital an average of 3 days, but occasionally longer if they have other medical complications that could slow their initial return home.

So think of what are the easiest things to reheat or prepare easily.

Post-Surgery

Others: Transportation home from the hospital.

The next crucial time that will arise for transportation needs are when it's time to begin your outpatient therapy, typically after 2-4 weeks after you're home.

This is where your therapy will continue and you will be getting around easier by then and ready for more aggressive therapy.

If by that time you're unable to drive yourself, then you will want to arrange for alternate options.

Equipment needs in the home *(examples: walker, bedside commode, shower chair, hospital bed, 3-in-1 commode, wheelchair etc.)*

Now I'm not saying you will have or even need *all* of these things,
but coordination of what is appropriate for your individual situation will be a discussion that you will want to have.

You can discuss this with your doctor, nurse and therapists while in the hospital as they are preparing for your return home.

When the equipment is delivered to your home, **you can ask the deliveryman to set it up or place it where you need it,** to alleviate you having to maneuver both yourself and equipment precariously around the house.

Others	Self
✓ Transportation from Hospital	✓ Meals and meal prep
✓ Equipment placed in the home	✓ Bed and toilet transfers
	✓ Icing for pain
	✓ Medication management

Self: Meals. Now hopefully you were able to prepare something that can easily be reheated before surgery (either homemade or store bought),
but other options to ponder are canned soups and easy to put together sandwiches.

Things that require very little prep, and little time on your feet, or even where you can be seated to prepare it.

Toilet transfers.

Safety is the key here.

So if you were not sent home with a bedside commode or a 3-in-1 commode that goes right over your toilet with arm rests, and if you did not already install grab bars by the toilet, then using your walker and backing up safely to the toilet will be key.

Even being able to use a countertop to support with your hands for standing and sitting, will be what you will need to do.

But NEVER rely or pull on a shower door or towel rack as support.

Those were not designed to take full body weight of pressure, and there are too many severe accidents as a result of them breaking and sending people flying.

Heed my caution.

It's *not* funny.

Bed transfers.

Getting in and out of bed will be a crucial task, but if you're unable to get into your own bed initially, then many people have resorted to a recliner chair or couch initially, to make life easier in the beginning.

Other options are using a belt or strap looped under the foot of your operated leg to assist it to swing up onto the bed.

This can be a great adaptation in the first few days, until the muscle have regained their strength to return to normal.

Medication management.

If you're not used to having a regular medication regimen, then **a pill box organizer can be a great help.** You can load it up for a week or even month at a time to take the guess work out of it.

Especially since you can be a little "loopy" and "foggy" in your mind due to pain and a very new situation that your body is adjusting to.

Icing for Pain Management.

In regards to icing, you might not grasp the reality and necessity of this just yet, but after surgery, **ice is going to be your *best friend!***

Trust me on this. ;)

Not only for pain reduction, but also to help decrease initial swelling, you're going to want ice easily at hand, multiple times a day.

So how can you prepare for this?

Easiest way would be to stock up on 2 or 3 gel ice packs before surgery, so you're already set to go once you get home and can rotate through them.

You'll want the gel kind, or crushed ice in a bag, or **Heck! even frozen peas,** so it can easily form over your knee for maximum contact and coverage. *See images below for examples.*

If you're solo at home and are still using a walker in the beginning, and the need for ice arrives, you'll need a means of carrying the ice with you to your landing spot (couch, bed, chair etc.).

So think of a bag you can sling around your arm or shoulder to carry the ice in temporarily, or some people even have a small bag or basket that they've purchased that attaches directly to their walker which can come in *very handy.*

Things to think about....:)

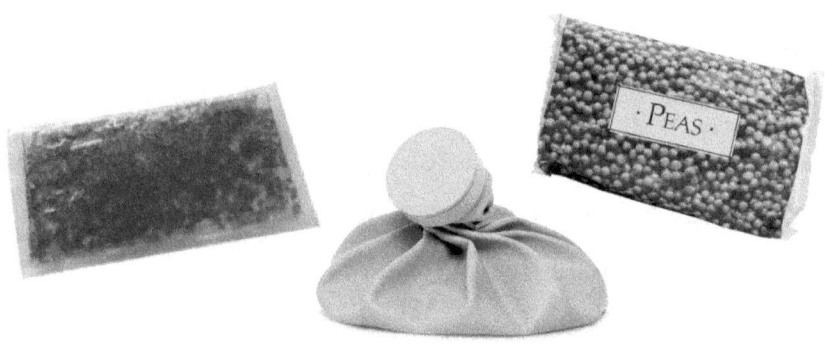

Final tips:

If you are very concerned about not having enough help after surgery, **discuss your options with your surgeon.**

They can help to facilitate a longer stay as needed at a rehab hospital or skilled nursing facility, until you recover enough to the point of being safe to care for yourself independently at home.

The hospital can make sure to connect you with their **Medical Social Worker** who can help with community resources and other considerations in what is called your *"Discharge Planning."*

Tackling Fear #5

Fear of the Financial Burden

As Sir Winston Churchill said,
"He who fails to plan is planning to fail."

There are many things to consider when it comes to the financial side of a major surgery like a knee replacement.

For most, this is a process and journey that is many months (even years) in the making and preparing. In order to help you ease the financial stresses.

Lets outline some of the areas that need to be considered:

> ✓ Your insurance plan: Do you have Medicare or private insurance? What are your deductibles that need to be met, if any? How is your plan set up? Knowing these answers in depth and

ahead of time, will help you plan for your portion of the costs.

✓ Your hospital stay: Expenses incurred during surgery, care received after surgery

✓ Your outpatient expenses: Physical therapy copays, equipment needs, follow up visits, etc.

✓ Additional considerations: Amount of time spent in the hospital post-op, pre-existing conditions, type of knee prosthetic implant and surgical approach, length of time in the operating room, unanticipated care or equipment needs etc.

On average in the U.S., a knee replacement surgery costs around $57,000, according to Medicare statistics, 2012.

But *your* portion will be greatly influenced by your insurance plan details.

So make sure to talk with your insurance representative and your surgeon about the expected costs and details of your insurance plan.

Other considerations will need to be planned for as well.

Including **time needed off work** that will affect your income, or if you **qualify for disability insurance,** which may be able help to supplement a portion of your income while you're recovering.

Plus extra out of pocket expenses for things that may not be covered by your insurance *(i.e. medical equipment for your home, home health therapy and nursing, hired caregivers etc.)*

To make it easier to visualize and plan, I've created a **Cheat Sheet** for you on the next page.
Photocopy and enlarge it.

Or you can visit
http://www.SuperiorKneeRehab.com/?p=366
and **print it out, full page.** *Get to it!*

[Cheat Sheet] Mapping Out The Finances

My Insurance Plan (write details while speaking with a representative)

Plan Name: Customer Service Phone #:

ID:

Valid until:

Deductible: Met or Not Met

Out of pocket maximum: Met or Not Met

Coinsurance:

Other details:

Hypothetical questions to ponder:

*Based on my insurance plan, if the average cost is $57,000, what is **my portion** and responsibility I can expect to owe?*

Do I qualify for Disability Insurance?   Yes   or   No
If yes, how much will this supplement for my income? $_____
How long will I receive these benefits?

If I'm currently working, how much would I need to save if I miss:

1 week of work: $_____

2 weeks of work: $_____

3 weeks of work: $_____

4 weeks of work: $_____

Other:

Considerations:
- Wages
- Bills
- Living necessities
- Hired help
- Copays/Doctor visits
- Transportation

© 2015 SuperiorKneeRehab.com

A major surgery like this can be so **rewarding and fulfilling** when it's all said and done, **but can also be overwhelming** if not fully discussed and investigated beforehand.

Make sure you're covering all of your bases to the best of your ability, and fearing the financial aspects of knee replacement surgery will soon begin to fade so you can **strategize and plan** for your best success.

I leave you with these wise words from Alexander Graham Bell,

"Before anything else, preparation is the key to success."

Conclusion

Thank you for spending this time with me as I've tried to explore and alleviate the top fears most people face when considering total knee replacement surgery.

I've tried to impart **practical knowledge and application** from both my personal experience as a physical therapist, and the best tips from all of my patient's over the years who have ***been in your shoes.***

Know that you are not alone.

Many have gone before you and are reaping the benefits and new-found freedom with their new knee(s), and many will follow after. :)

Here's to your best knees!

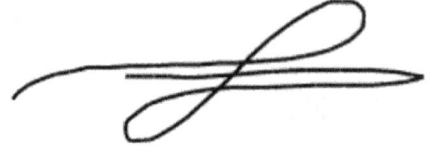

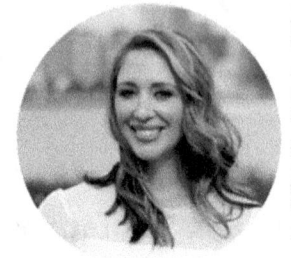

~*Dr. Melody Stevens, PT, DPT*

Physical Therapist, Founder SuperiorKneeRehab.com

P.S. I'd love to have you join me on our Facebook page for weekly tips to give you *less knee pain* and inspiration so you're living every day to the fullest.

Visit http://www.facebook.com/SuperiorKneeRehab

P.P.S. I'd love to have you join me for my latest free online training to continue to help your knees. Details on the next page.

Top 5 Critical Exercises Before Knee Replacement Surgery

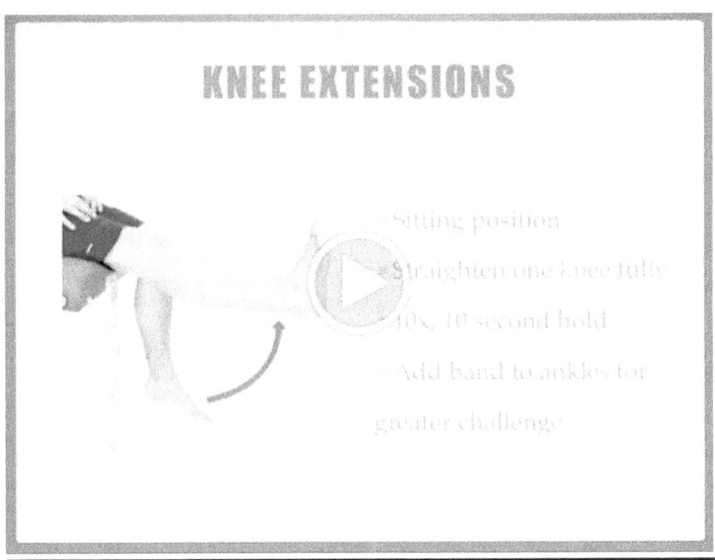

- The top **5 most critical exercises** to strengthen and stretch the right muscles, giving you **better joint mobility, less knee pain** and knowing exactly **how to be prepared** for a future knee replacement surgery.

- You can **get started right away** with these 5 targeted exercises knowing the proper technique and form, and how to progress yourself for continued improvement and ultimately, **less knee pain,** whether you have surgery or not.

Go to this link to **reserve your spot** for this free training at

FreeKneeVideos.com

www.ingramcontent.com/pod-product-compliance
Lightning Source LLC
Chambersburg PA
CBHW070746180526
45168CB00004B/1549